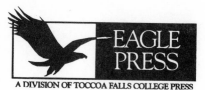

A DIVISION OF TOCCOA FALLS COLLEGE PRESS

ISBN: 1-885729-16-2

Printed by Toccoa Falls College Press
P.O. Box 800067
Toccoa Falls, GA 30598

Forward

Bent...But Not Broken is a story of love and hope. It captures the moment....the shock of discovering that your child has cancer...the kneeling beside her bed in prayer that God's grace will be with her...the subsequent prayers of help and hope...the memories of words spoken before and after surgery...the alien experience of treatments and all the good and bad that they incorporate...the fears, the anguish, the questions...the miracle of modern medicine and the blessed ones that practice that profession...the encouragement of friends...the growth of family unity...and the confidence that God is with us always.

Coming Soon is the only poem that was written outside the time we discovered the tumor. We felt it appropriate to include in the book because it describes the exuberating joy of discovering that our baby was on the way and the wonderful experience of her birth. Some poems are our prayers. *Daddy, Daddy* was inspired by Alyson when she awoke in intensive care to see her Daddy standing over her crying. She merely said, "Daddy, Daddy, please don't cry," and went back to sleep. Alyson asked her daddy to write *Little Star* because of the florescent, glow-in-the-dark stars that decorated the door to the bathroom in her hospital room. Many of the poems are written from Alyson's perspective and we feel they capture the experiences she had during initial diagnosis, her hospital stay and subsequent chemo-treatments.

Our confidence is that Alyson will defeat cancer, however, we are also painfully aware that others do not; thus, *What If The Valley Were Too Deep* was written in memory of those that do not win the battle.

Our hopes are that everyone who reads this book will be touched by our experience and will come to know God's powerful and saving grace. It is our prayer that in all of life's struggles may you be bent...but not broken.

Terri Queen
Alyson's Mom

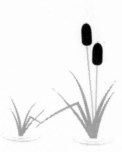

To All Cancer Victims

May the fabric of your struggle be woven
with the same threads of courage and
determination
used by our 5-year old daughter

ALYSON TAYLOR QUEEN

to defeat her cancer January 1997 through August
1997
and to whom
this book of celebration is dedicated.

W. Patrick Queen
Teresa L. Queen

Our most special thanks are given to
Our Holy Father,
Our God Most High,
For His Peace, Patience and Prosperity
During this struggle.

Through all things He has loved us,
Nurtured us and been faithful.

His healing power and grace is immeasurable!!

We give Him the praise and glory
And honor Him for His goodness in
Healing our Daughter.

We are forever indebted to His instruments
And their faithfulness to be used of God
In the healing of our precious little girl!

We offer you our deepest gratitude
And heartfelt love.
We express our thanks through
The Message of this collection of poetry,

Bent...
but not Broken!
A Family's Victory Over Cancer...
Through The Grace Of God!

Our love and appreciation go to:

Dr. Jamison Satterfield
Dr. Orren Beaty
Dr. Eric Walburgh
Dr. R. J. Waller
Dr. Eric F. Kuehn
The Staff at The Ruth & Billy Graham Children's Health Center
The Staff at The Pediatric Outpatient Unit,
Mission Memorial Hospital
The Hospital Staff at Mountain Radiation Oncology, P.A.
Laurel Wanner, Child Life Specialist
Anne Manke, R.N.
Vanessa Justice, R.N.
Emily Clark, R.N.
Melanie Clark, R.N.
Kimberly Delk, R.N.
Deborah Isley, Hospital Chaplain
Sylvia G. Faulk
Barbara and Ted Van Thullenar and
The Friends of Santa Claus
The Staff at The Lewis Rathbun Wellness Center
Clayton Baptist Church, Clayton, Georgia
First Baptist Church of Mocksville, North Carolina
Liberty Baptist Church, Tiger, Georgia
Lakemont Baptist Church, Lakemont, Georgia
First Methodist Children's V.B.S, Clayton, Georgia
All the many friends that lifted up continual prayers that
our precious daughter might be healed
All the generous donors to
The Alyson Taylor Queen Cancer Fund

And, of course, Josie!

God Bless You!

A Special Thanks

This book represents many hours of tears, anguish, laughter and pain. The fruits of our love and labor are best represented in the special art and illustrations of a very talented man...

Broderick Crawford

We give him our heartfelt thanks and offer him our unending joy in celebrating with us the health of our sweet child...

To Broderick

A truer friend can never be
Than one that walks life's paths with me,
Who shares the bitter and the best
And helps me face life's toughest test;
And you my friend are tried and true...
With many thanks, this book's for you!

Pat, Terri & Alyson

Table of Contents

Coming Soon

It started out as heartburn
Or a severe touch of gas;
But after several days of misery,
It had not begun to pass.

So, off we went together
Through the doctor's door that day
To find out a special joy
Would be coming soon our way.

And, so for nine long months
That stretched out like eternity,
I waited patiently on your dear Mom
To deliver you to me.

Yes, I would be the proudest Dad
With the biggest smile upon my face.
For you would be the grandest child
Ever born to the human race.

The days they quickly hastened now
The "blessed event" was close at hand.
Your Mom had grown so large
That it was hard for her to stand.

But, with all the strength and courage
That she could muster on that morn,
We set out for the hospital;
Today, you would be born!

And in a very special room
Where miracles come true...
The doctor said, "Push, I see the head..."
And your Mom gave life to you.

Now, all my life I've been told
How special that moment can be;
But I never knew joy, nor life, nor love
'Til they handed you to me.

And in that first meeting
As I gazed into your eyes,
I thanked the Lord, our Father,
For you, my special prize.

For not for who I am
Nor my plans of what to be,
But for the grace of God
Has He entrusted you to me.

And so, my darling daughter,
Should this verse you ever see,
May this you know, where 'ere you go,
YOU MEAN THE WORLD TO ME!!!

All my love,

Daddy
June 15, 1993

Instead

I must have awakened a thousand times
The thoughts racing through my head.
My daughter's facing cancer;
Why can't it be me instead?

What a beautiful child; what a wonderful laugh;
What an impish, little smile on her face.
She's got no idea what lies ahead...
Please, Lord, let me take her place.

I'll endure all that must be done,
I promise I won't complain.
Just spare my child all this horrible grief...
Please don't let her feel any pain.

I know it seems like a lot to ask,
To let me be the one
To suffer and wrestle with this malady,
But you'd have done the same for your Son.

Christ put His faith, His trust in you,
He knew that you'd see Him through.
So, I'm going to believe that all I need
Is to do the same thing too.

So into Thy hands I place my faith
And the life of my daughter too.
And now we're counting on you, dear God
To help us see this through.

For when we emerge on the other side
We'll praise you forevermore,
For our faith will be stronger, our love secure;
And our daughter's health restored.

January 28, 1997

Daddy, Daddy

Daddy, Daddy, please don't cry.
I know I look tired and weak,
But you must listen when I speak
And wipe the tears from your eye.

Daddy, Daddy, please don't cry.
I know you don't really understand,
But stay by me and hold my hand
And I promise I won't die.

Daddy, Daddy, please don't cry.
I'm not well, but I'm getting better.
I'll follow their instructions to the letter
I'll try not to ask why.

Daddy, Daddy, please don't cry.
The pain is really not so bad.
I hate to see you look so sad;
You must promise me that you'll try!

Daddy, Daddy, it's okay to cry.
I know you're trying to be brave.
But don't worry, my life we'll save
Together, we'll reach for the sky!!

January 30, 1997

Live Long

Tumor.

Terrible.   Traumatic. Tumultuous.

Cancer.

Cold-blooded.   Calculating.   Contemptuous.
Caustic.   Catastrophic!

Life?

LONG.

My feelings are mixed. Blended.
Focused on one central thought.

WIN...AT ANY COST!!!

Beat. Annihilate.
Destroy this wretched demon that has taken control.

Robbing me of my childhood.
Destroying my dreams.
Vanishing my hopes.
But **I WILL WIN!!!**

I will fight and regain control of my life,
My thoughts, my emotions.

For I will be...ME
And nothing can take over me unless I will it.
I will not give in...For I shall be well and....

LIVE LONG!

January 30, 1997

My Greatest Day

They brought me to the hospital.
They said that I was sick;
But Granddaddy said, "Don't worry!
You won't miss a lick,"

Of playing with my puzzles,
My computer games and toys;
I'll soon be back to romping
With the other girls and boys.

I know that something terrible
Is growing inside of me;
I'm not sure just what that means,
But I know it shouldn't be.

So, I'll listen to my doctors
And the orders from my nurse.
I'll try to do just what they say
To get rid of this deadly curse.

I'll let the doctors poke and prod;
Through it all, I will be brave;
I know they'll do what's best for me
If my life they're going to save.

Mom and Dad will be there too
To help me fight this thing
For I've got a lot more life to live;
I've got a lot more songs to sing.

Yes, my grandest triumph lies ahead,
My greatest day is yet to be!
I'll hug my nurses, shake the doctors' hand
And shout, "Praise God...I'm cancer free!!!

January 30, 1997

7

One More Day

Lord,
Give me courage for just one more day.
Give me courage to travel life's highway.
Give me courage to finish what I've begun.
Give me courage to pray, "Thy will be done."

Lord,
Give me faith for just one more day.
Give me faith to trust in what others say.
Give me faith to move mountains or to dry up the sea.
Give me faith to believe that Christ died for me.

Lord,
Give me trust for just one more day.
Give me trust when things don't go my way.
Give me trust when my skies turn dark and gray.
Give me trust in you for just one more day.

Lord,
Give me strength for just one more day.
Give me strength to stand firm and never sway.
Give me strength for the battles I'll face each day.
Give me strength, Oh Lord, how I need you today.

Lord,
Give me peace for just one more day.
Give me peace to know how I should pray.
Give me peace in my soul that can't be taken away.
Give me your peace, dear Lord, just enough for today.

Lord,
Give me love for just one more day.
Give me more than enough so I might give it away.
Give me love to engulf those that pass my way.
Give me love that abides for more than today.

Lord,
Give me courage and the faith I receive;
May you grant me the trust and the strength to believe
That the peace and the love that fills me today
Will meet all of my needs for just one more day.

January 31, 1997

Friend Or Foe?

Cold, slender, sullen; towering above,
Shows no emotion, gives no love.
It's my shadow wherever I go
Never says yes; never says no.

Stands by my bed from dark 'til dawn.
If I go to the toilet, it tags along.
I'm not sure yet if he's friend or foe,
But I know he follows wherever I go.

My pole's my sentry; he's a stand-up guy.
He's heard me laugh, he listens when I cry.
Alone at night, he's hears my screams,
He knows my doubts, my fears, my dreams.

We're fighting a war; there can be no truce.
My buddy holds the ammo of "super juice."
Out of the bag and down through the line
We fire our salvoes, one drip at a time.

He's always with me. I know now he's my friend,
And together we'll fight to the bitter end;
'Cause my buddy's beside me through thick or thin.
**We will fight this cancer and
We will win!!!**

February 1, 1997

10

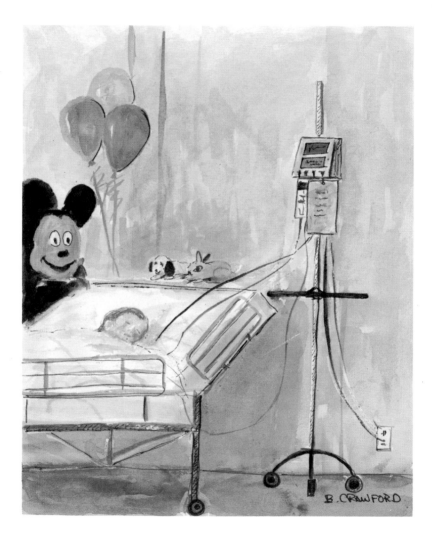

Little Star

Twinkle, twinkle little star
Hung upon my bathroom door...
You're the brightest one by far,
Shine on me forevermore.

You're like a diamond in the sky,
Heaven's most wondrous light;
Hung above the world so high,
My guardian through the night.

So, twinkle, twinkle my little star,
I know you cannot stay,
But when you leave, please don't go far;
Come back and light my way!

February 2, 1997

Don't Give Up

I know this must be overwhelming
for Daddy's five year old.
Just a few days ago,
the biggest thing you had to think about
Was what to have for lunch.
Now you must suffer through the pain, the nausea,
The phone ringing in your hospital room
Just after you've finally fallen asleep.

My Little Darling, we've begun this journey
That leads back to health, happiness
And a wonderful life with Mommy and me.
It won't be easy!
You will get sick so that you can get well.
But you will get well!!!
You must believe that
and fight with all your growing power.
Whatever you face, you are not alone...
God holds you in His Hands.
So, remember, no matter what happens,
you will be okay...
Just don't give up.

February 2, 1997

13

If I Just Call On You

My life seems dark and desperate;
Sorrow surrounds my soul.
My world's been blown apart;
What can make me whole?

You've promised that You'll love me,
So hope comes shining through;
You're always there to guide me,
If I just call on You.

The road seems long and perilous;
There's danger everywhere.
My heart is saddened, broken-down,
Laden with despair.

But You are there with open arms,
You know just what to do
And I am never left alone,
If I just call on You.

If I just call on You, my Lord,
You answer every prayer.
You fill my life with lasting joy,
Your sweet peace fills the air.

My troubles seem to vanish,
They're gone like morning dew;
And day breaks fresh and glorious,
When I just call on You.

So, forgive me, my Father,
When I doubt what You can do,
And I try to make it on my own
Without consulting You.

Oh, teach me this lesson, Lord,
Write upon my heart so true:
You grant me love and joy and peace...
When I just call on You.

February 4, 1997

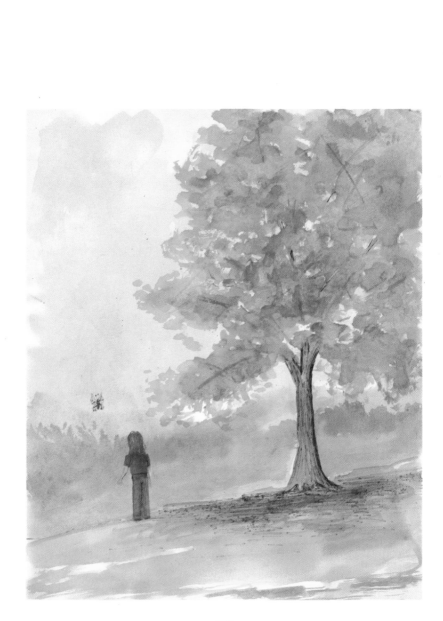

Mighty Oaks

Like a giant oak that stands tall against the sky;
Roots like thirsty straws gathering nourishment when it's dry;
There is no storm or peril that can fell so grand a tree
And in this work of nature, there's a lesson for you and me.

From just a tiny acorn planted in the deepest, richest sands
Grows this towering testimony to the majesty of God's hands.
A single, little bud that comes bursting forth in spring
Filled with all God's creatures, their melodies they sing;

And with each passing season as the years may come and go,
This once small, tender sapling into a mighty oak does grow.
Its powerful, gnarling limbs arch gracefully toward the sun
Offering shade and sweet repose for those whose work is done.

As centuries come with each new age, the oak is stalwart still.
Its majesty and grandeur, the elements cannot kill.
This warrior survives all pestilence as it reaches above,
And each of us will thrive and grow when grounded in God's love.

So when life's burdens weigh you down or you're feeling all alone,
Remember little acorns into mighty oaks have grown.
Just plant your tiny seed of faith in the Master's Holy sod
And you will grow, like mighty oaks, to touch the face of God.

February 5, 1997

How Can This Be?

As I sit here by her bedside, I try hard not to cry.
I fight the urge inside me to scream and ask God, "Why?"
Why, oh God, choose my little girl,
The apple of my eye?
What purpose could this misery serve; oh, why not pass her by?

What could she have possibly done? Or, Father was it me?
That brought this dreadful cancer, this unending misery.
She's such a perfect angel.
How can this truly be?
So, if you really love us, Lord, remove this malady.

For we know you have the power, Lord;
It's well within your might
To prove us victorious, to help us win this fight;
To clear away the dark clouds of this never-ending night;
To help us see more clearly your glorious, healing light.

We'll try hard not to doubt you, we'll try hard to understand.
We'll try to believe through all of this,
It's part of your Master Plan.
We will not falter in our faith; we'll trust you all we can.
We know there is no power that can snatch us from your hand.

So, hear our prayer, dear Father, grant us your peace today.
Heal our darling baby girl, wipe her tears away.
Grant us your strength and power sufficient for this day
Enfold us in your loving arms; draw close to us and stay.

February 7, 1997

I'm Only A Five-Year Old

I was awake all last night, tossing and turning.
My body aches, my side hurts, my tummy's churning.
I wish the pain would leave me so I could get some rest.
I need Mommy's sweet kiss, her touch of tenderness.

I'm only a five year old...I just want to play;
But I'm told I'll have to fight this cancer again today.
I wish I wasn't so tired and didn't feel so bad.
Why do Mommy and Daddy have to look so sad?

Maybe I can have pizza again today for lunch?
I hope this medicine they're giving me doesn't hurt a bunch.
The doctors and the nurses are very nice to me,
But I'm tired of all this attention; I wish they'd let me be.

I've been poked and stuck with needles and every time I cry.
I've heard that cancer can cause people to die.
I need to be like Mommy, she's so brave and bold,
But that's a lot to ask of a five-year old.

Today, they operated on me and took my kidney out;
I'm trying to smile and be happy; I'm trying not to pout.
But I'm so tired and cranky; I'm shivering and I'm cold.
This is a lot to endure, when you're only a five-year old.

February 14, 1997

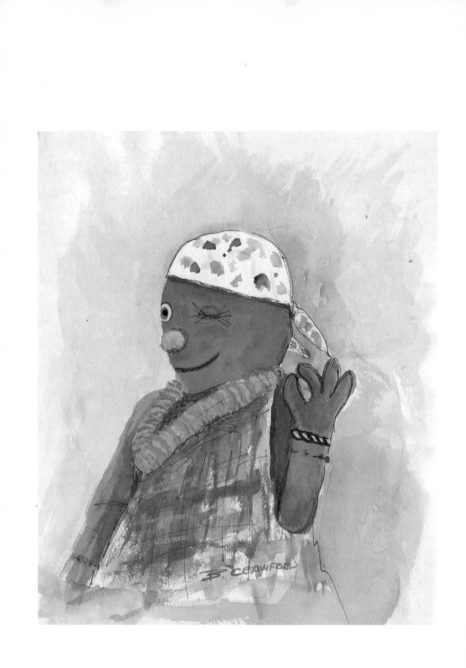

My Friend Josie

We know roses are red and violets are posies.
Did you know my best friend at the hospital
Was a little girl named Josie?

Now Josie was sharp in ways you might think
And I didn't mind that her skin was dark pink.

She wore the same dress each day she was there.
But it was really quite lovely with her bright yellow hair.

We'd laugh, we'd chuckle and wildly cavort;
Josie showed me where they put in her port.

She told me about what the doctors would do.
She even let me shine her turquoise shoes.

Each day Josie prepared me for what lay ahead
She'd talk with me sweetly as she sat on my bed.

She said the doctors would take my tumor out
And I should be brave and try not to pout.

So, I promised Josie I would not make a peep,
When I got the shot that would make me sleep.

After my operation I was brought to intensive care;
When I opened my eyes, my friend Josie was there.

She smiled down at me with those bright green eyes
And the next thing that happened was quite a surprise.

You see, puppets aren't real people;
At least that's what we think,
But I know I saw my friend Josie give me a wink.

So, I don't care if I live to be a hundred and three;
I'll never forget our time together, just Josie and me!

February 27, 1997

21

E.R.

My port was in, the tumor out,
The cancer gone.
There could be no doubt.

So pack my bags and take my hand,
It's time to blow
This popsicle stand.

But "Wait," said the doctor,
"Don't start the celebration;
You've got to have some external radiation."

External radiation?
Now, what can that be?
They're gonna shoot gamma rays inside of me.

So they rolled me down the hall
In a rickety wheelchair.
It seemed to take forever for us to get there.

They took me into
The treatment room
It was cold and damp, a place of gloom.

The nurse asked me to climb onto the table.
Mommy had to help
'Cause I wasn't able.

They told me to lie still,
Try not to even blink.
Then the doctor drew on me with permanent ink.

He made little lines and dots that he could see,
But I said,
"Daddy doesn't like anyone writing on me"

I lay really still
For what seemed like days.
I wanted to leave and go out and play.

But the nurses were just as nice as could be,
And each day when we finished
They gave presents to me.

At last it was time,
We had done the simulation;
So the doctor began my external radiation.

Everyone would leave,
Mommy'd kiss me on my cheek.
They'd all stand outside, at the monitor they'd peek.

The machine would hum,
But I'd lie very still,
Trying not to shiver whenever I got a chill.

Next thing I know, the machine flips around;
Taking pictures of my backside,
But I didn't make a sound.

Then the beeping stops and the nurse comes in;
She says I'm doing great,
So let's try it again.

I lie really still like they say I should.
I do the best I can
To be brave and good.

I really don't understand what they're doing to me;
But I know when we're done,
I'll be cancer free.

Yes, I long for the day of my great celebration,
And I'm thankful I'm done
With this external radiation.

February 27, 1997

23

If It's Tuesday

Pack my bag and away we go,
If it's Tuesday, it must be chemo.

Grab my stuff, let's jump in the car.
I'm glad we don't have to travel far.

Just pack some toys for me to play.
I won't be back 'til late today.

The car climbs the mountains, it chugs along.
Mommy and I sing my "Wild One" song.

She lathers my port with the numbing cream.
When she peels it off, I cry and scream.

The nurses all laugh and talk with me
Trying to distract me so I won't see

All the tests and procedures they have to do;
They take my blood and my urine, too.

I try to be brave, I try not to cry.
I try to look the doctor right in the eye.

I tell him a joke or a funny Disney line.
He tells my parents everything's just fine.

I know they say I have nothing to fear,
So I let the nurse stick that thing in my ear.

Three little beeps means she is done,
And I can go back to having more fun.

Playing with the games and toys that are there.
This chemo I'm taking makes me lose my hair.

But I never laugh, chuckle or snort
When it's time for the nurse to access my port.

For when this happens, it's the most serious part
As the doctor listens to my pounding heart.

The nurse takes the line, now I feel sick.
I try not to whimper when I feel the small prick.

She shoots the drugs through the access line;
Then I'm stylin' and profilin', feelin' just fine.

For in a flash of an instant, the ordeal is over,
And I'm ready to romp and roll through the clover.

You see takin' this chemo is no big deal
If I wanna make sure this cancer I'll kill.

So, week after week, I'll be back I know
'Cause if it's Tuesday, it must be chemo.

March 1, 1997

What's Up Doc?

I went to see my doctor just the other day.
Had a pain in my side, what it was I couldn't say.
So I opened up the door, stepped into the waiting room,
The nurse said, "Have a seat, the doc will see you soon."

So, I grabbed up some toys and I began to play
Hopin' this exam wouldn't keep me here all day;
In a matter of minutes, who should appear,
But the nurse and my doctor in full exam gear.

Now he's a hubba-hubba guy - with real sex appeal,
My pediatrician, Dr. Jamie Satterfield.
For he's the only guy that I've come to know
That I'll let examine me from my head to my toes.

I jumped up on the table to begin my examination.
He pushed and he poked and with a look of consternation,
He turned to my parents and he had them sit down.
He said, "We're going to need to get an ultra sound."

We left his office, just drove a little way
To another building where they could do the X-ray.
In a flash, it was over and I was ready to ride.
How little did we know what was growing inside.

Dr. Satterfield talked with his nurse for a while
Then he set down with me and he flashed his big smile.
"I've looked at your X-ray," he said without humor,
"I believe that knot in your side is a Wilm's tumor."

"What's a Wilm's tumor?" we asked; but could not believe the answer.
My left kidney was being held hostage by a childhood cancer.
Mommy began to cry and Daddy did too;
I didn't know just what I should do.

But my doctor knew the answer; he knew what we needed.
Said follow his advice and see that his instructions were heeded:
"Find a pediatric oncologist and pediatric surgeon;
And do it right away, for it is really quite urgent!"

They say I'm pretty smart for a five year old
And I'm so very thankful we did what we were told.
Yes, my kidney's gone, but the tumor is too.
I'm still fighting this cancer, but you can bet when I'm through

There's one special guy I want to see while I'm still five
To thank him for his part in keeping me alive.
And if it won't make him an emotional wreck,
I'll give him A BIG KISS AND A HUG around the neck!
I Love You!
Alyson Taylor Queen

March 19, 1997

Hand Of God

It was just another Saturday night
As we started up the stairs,
How little did I know
Of the horror waiting there.

We gathered all her Barbie dolls
And placed them on the floor.
We would send Barbie on her date
Or to the senior prom once more.

I sat down behind her
Although that's not my usual place.
I prefer to sit across from her
To see her smiling face.

Those big brown eyes, those chocolate drops
That melt a mother's heart...
How could I know what lay ahead,
The suffering about to start.

My darling, innocent 5-year old
Lay snuggled up next to me.
I began to rub her tummy
When I felt the abnormality.

A hard knot beneath her ribs...
That felt like an old door knob,
And I might never have found it
If not for the Hand of God.

I rubbed for what seemed like hours.
I would poke and push and prod;
And all the time I rubbed her side
It was really the Hand of God.

God's healing hand was already at work.
Though my thoughts were void of humor,
A sickening feeling overcame me;
My daughter had a cancerous tumor.

Yes, I thank God that He hears my prayers,
As through this world I trod,
I'll praise His name forevermore
And give thanks for the Hand of God.

For I would not give in to fear
Though terror gripped my soul.
I would pray that the Hand of God
Would heal her, make her whole.

God would provide the surgeon
With a sure and steady hand.
Together we could beat this cancer
So, again, my child would stand...

Tall and proud and full of life
Walking next to me
And I would kneel and thank my God
That my child is cancer free.

April 4, 1997

My Little Girl With Eyes So Brown

My little girl with eyes so brown
Who never cries, who seldom frowns.
Your life's been changed; turned upside down
And there's nothing I can do.

You seem so weak, so frail, so small;
You hardly eat anything these days at all.
I always come running anytime you call
To see what I can do.

I hate this blasted chemotherapy.
I hate to see you suffer such misery.
I wish instead of you, it could be me.
Now, that's something I could do.

But, we both know God doesn't work that way;
So we'll have to see it through day to day.
I promise by your side I will always stay
To do what I can do.

So, my dearest daughter, hold your chin up high.
Fight the fight that will cause this cancer to die;
And together as a family we will reach for the sky,
And I'll love you in all that you do.

April 12, 1997

The House With A Giant Heart

Well off the beaten path, tucked neatly in the woods
Stands a special place dedicated to doing the greatest good.
For all who cross this threshold and there in sign their name,
They'll not depart this house with a heart and ever be the same.

For no matter what your burden
Or the woes that have brought you here,
You'll feel the love and compassion of the volunteers who care,
About your waking moments or your night of restful sleep,
For the friends you make at the Rathbun House
Are friends you'll always keep.

So, when disease attacks your body or that of a family member
Just close your eyes, take a cleansing breath;
This thought you must remember:
The journey to wellness that lies ahead
Might begin with a rocky start,
But you're never alone with this house as your home...

The House With the Giant Heart!!

May 9, 1997

The Head Badge Of Courage

Walking down the hallway
My eyes peek into each room
Expecting to see deep despair
And overwhelming gloom.

For in each room on this hospital floor
Are God's most courageous ones,
These little children fighting cancer,
Our daughters and our sons.

It doesn't matter what their age
For cancer knows no bounds.
It creeps into their little lives
And never makes a sound.

They fight and fight with all their might.
You'd think they'd get discouraged,
But none give in and each proudly wears
Their unique head badge of courage.

At first it seems a little strange
For a child that is so small
To run, to play, to laugh and cry
With a head completely bald.

But as a parent with a hairless child
My heart, it swells with pride;
For I know that her badge of courage
Is a sign of the fight inside.

This battle in my daughter must rage on
If this war we're going to win.
We'll fight this enemy toe to toe;
We will fight to the bitter end.

Along the way we'll have our ups and downs.
We will do our best not to become discouraged,
For we take great pride in our daughter's fight
And her beautiful head badge of courage.

April 1997

Power Of Prayer

The journey had begun, to where we did not know,
But listening to the doctors, we knew we had a long way to go.
We might still be wandering through the valley of despair
If not for God's people and the power of their prayer.

Oh, the power of prayer is a wondrous, glorious thing.
It can set the captive heart free once again to sing.
It can lift the burdened soul up, though loaded down with care.
You must never underestimate the mighty power of prayer.

For the Father has instructed those called by his name
To put our faith and trust in Him, His promises to claim.
We can carry our burdens to His throne
And prayerfully leave them there;
Our lives are changed, our burdens lifted
Through the power of our prayer.

As we have fought this battle, we have never been alone,
For the prayers of His people have brought us to the throne.
They've carried us to Jesus, His grace and love to share,
And we now know God's healing touch
Through the power of their prayer.

So when life's storm clouds gather and your heart is full of pain,
Just pray to the Father and like a gentle rain,
He'll wash away your anguish, He'll vanish every care;
He'll grant your every heart's desire
Through the power of your prayer.

April 14, 1997

35

And In This Corner....

The crowd was nervous, restless, as they began to shuffle in
For the fight of the century was about to begin.
The challenger was tiny; a small and delicate child.
The champion flexed his muscles and the crowd went wild.

This would be so easy, not much of a fight
The champion would hardly break a sweat, his work would be light.
For over in the corner was this weak, uninspiring thing;
She wouldn't stand a chance when she stepped into the ring.

The announcer grabbed the microphone, a hush fell upon the crowd.
He stepped into the center ring; his booming voice so loud
As he screamed, "Ladies and gentlemen, we're mighty glad you came
And after this evening's bout, you won't leave here the same."

"Now, in this corner's our challenger, I'm told she's only five.
If our champion has his way with her, she won't leave here alive.
I'm sure you know this beastly one, though he goes by many names;
For in every fight he seeks to win, to cripple and to maim.

Our champion cares not who he fights; their sex, their health, their age;
And very few defeat him unless they can match his rage.
So let's see what lies ahead tonight; does this child have the answer?
Can she defeat the mighty one...the champion known as "Cancer"?

The bell rings, the champion moves, deadly without a sound.
He lunges, as he throws his punches, her body he begins to pound.
First with pokes and needles; then her kidney they remove.
His punches are relentless; his point he's trying to prove.

36

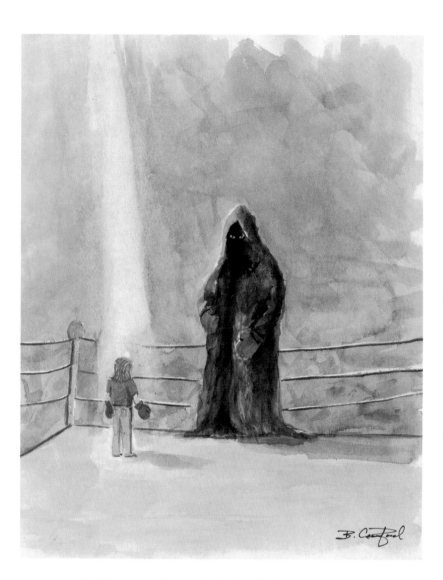

He'll keep pounding on her body, a little more each day
In hopes that she'll give in to him and let him have his way.
He must be the victor, for when all's said and done;
Chalk one up for cancer, he's claimed another one.

But wait a minute sports' fans,
Can you believe your eyes?
This little gal's a fighter,
She's refusing to die.
She won't give in to cancer,
She's fighting with all her might,
And I am here to tell you, friends,
This is not cancer's lucky night.

She's punched him in the stomach,
She's pounding back his ears.
This could be the worst licking
Cancer's taken in many years.
She's really quite a battler,
This "cancer-fightin' machine,"
This tiny, courageous champion,
Alyson Taylor Queen.

So, if you face an upcoming bout with this rarely beaten foe,
Remember this little child of God and in your heart you'll know
To have beaten this champion by herself was surely too great a task;
But in her corner was the Heavenly Host...and all she did was ask!

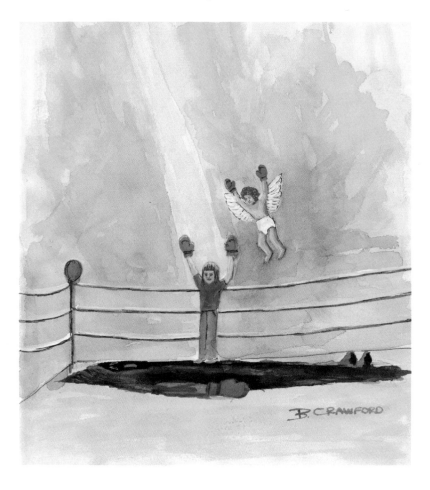

April 10, 1997

All Is Well

Another day has come and gone
And with the setting sun
We're one day closer to our goal
The battle's almost won.

We're one fight closer to the time
When this cancer will be beaten.
We can almost taste the victory now
A taste that seems to sweeten.

Every sight that meets the eye
To everyone we'll tell
The victory now is close at hand
And soon all will be well.

Our Saviour holds us near to him.
Our burdens alone He bears.
He lifts us up in our darkest hour
And removes our worldly cares.

He keeps us safe from all other harm
Though He casts no magic spell.
In Christ we find such sweet repose,
In Him we know all is well.

So hold us close, dear Jesus,
Our Lord, Emanuel;
And we shall praise your healing power
For in you...all is well!

We thank you for your saving grace
And all the blessings that you give.
We thank you most for our precious gift,
Our daughter who still lives.

So with each day that comes, dear Lord,
May your message to others we tell.
May we lead them to know that eternal peace
Is in you...and, all is well.

Easter 1997

What If The Valley Were Too Deep?

What if the valley were too deep?
>   The journey far too long...
What if we give all we have
>   But sing no victor's song?

What for all our loved ones
>   Who struggle with us each day
When we've gone to meet our Father
>   And they're left behind to stay...

To wrestle with the pain and grief,
>   The lonely agony?
What can we say before we go
>   That will help them to see?

Do not mourn for us, for now
>   In Christ, there's rest and sleep,
And He was with us all the way
>   Though the valley was too deep.

We may not sing our earthly songs
>   We may not run the race
For we've been called to our glorious reward
>   In the Saviour's abiding place.

Cry not for us, dear Mothers.
>   Blessed Fathers, do not weep.
For the Saviour carried us in His arms
>   When the valley was too deep.

We thank you for your undying love,
>   The sacrifices given,
And we shall await the day
>   When at last we meet in heaven.

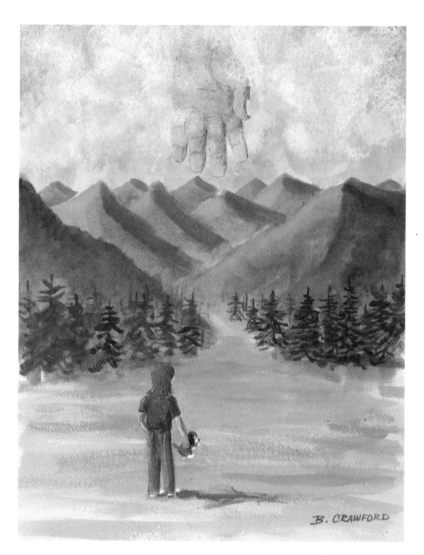

And then, at last, you too will know our Lord's promise, He did keep.
The Father's love will see you through,
When the valley is too deep.

April 5, 1997

43

Bent...But Not Broken

Into such a little life, the storm of cancer came;
The thunder of catastrophe, the tears of a torrential rain.
How could God the Father allow this calamity?
Why did cancer choose our little girl; oh, why couldn't it be me?

I thought of all the promises the Bible gives to us;
How we're to put our faith in Him, in Him we place our trust.
For He promised we could move mountains, if we only believe,
But how we could defeat this cancer was hard to conceive.

Our world had been shattered, broken apart by this storm.
Our spirits were discouraged, our hearts were forlorn;
The Father said, "Fear not, my child, though you may be heartbroken,
Though the howling winds of cancer blow, you will be
Bent....but not Broken."

Bent...but not Broken...the special message of God's Son,
"For I have come to conquer, in all things to overcome.
This message I give to you, my child, though oft it go unspoken;
Through storm or gale or life's raging winds, you might be
Bent...but not Broken."

So, no matter what you face in life, no matter how great the task;
The Father will draw near to you, if you but only ask.
The promise that He gave to you is not merely just a token;
In all life's storms, he'll see you through; you might be
Bent...but not Broken.

And so, dear Father, we implore you to see us through this gale.
We know that through your mercy against this cancer we will prevail.
We find in you our solace, we take comfort in words bespoken.
We know that as a child of yours, we shall be
Bent...But Never Broken.

April 5, 1997

45

To arrange a speaking engagement
or to order additional copies
of this book
call
1-706-782-1991
or contact
W. Patrick Queen
c/o The Poet's Porch
P.O. Box 1947
Clayton, GA 30525